NATURALWAYS TO TREAT& PREVENT FIBROIDS

Dr BAYO

TABLE OF CONTENTS

Overview on uterine fibroid

Most women have benign (non-cancerous) developed known as fibroids in their womb (uterus). Many fibroids are tiny and don't cause any problems. They are usually seen by chance. Depending on where fibroids are located, they may bring about period pain, heavy menstrual bleeding or other symptoms.

There are various ways to cure fibroids. The most appropriate cure will greatly rely on a woman's personal circumstances – such as whether she would still like to bear children.

Fibroids are comprises of muscle cells and connective tissue. Their size, shape and location vary. Fibroids are principally categorized based on where they are in the womb:

- Directly under the lining of the womb (submucosal fibroids)

- In the wall of the womb (intramural fibroids)

- On the outer wall of the womb (subserosal fibroids)

- In the cervix (cervical fibroids)

In the connective tissue close to the womb (intraligamentary fibroids) Reseachers estimate that about 40 to 80% of all women have fibroids. Most of the fibroids are very tiny, and many women never notice that they have them. Fibroids only once in a while cause symptoms, but it's very difficult to say exactly how often, and likely they are to do so.

It's also difficult to predict how a fibroid will go on to develop: Fibroids develop to various sizes and at other speeds. Some fibroids and their associated symptoms hardly change despite not having cure. Other fibroids develop larger, and the symptoms get bad over time. Symptoms may also slowly go away on their own.

Fibroids normally reduced after a woman has reached menopause, and then the symptoms will almost disappear as well. Having hormone therapy for menopause symptoms may reduced fibroids from shrinking in most cases. Then the fibroid symptoms wouldn't go away either.

Chapter One

BRIEF HISTORY ON FIBROIDS

Fibroids are known, hormone-relying on, benign uterine tumors. They can make significant morbidity and the symptoms relying broadely on their size. The purpose of this reaearch was to describe the natural history of fibroids and identify factors that may affect their development

 However, this is a retrospective longitudinal research of premenopausal women who were diagnosed with uterine fibroids on ultrasound examination. Almost every woman underwent at least two transvaginal ultrasound scans that were all performed by a single operator. Fibroids were calculated in three perpendicular planes and the mean diameter was measured. The size and position of each person fibroid was assessed and recorded on a computerized database. The volume of each fibroid was measured using the formula for a sphere.

A total of 122 women were included in the research. Their median age at the initial examination was 40 (range, 27-48) years. Seventy-two (59.0%) were nulliparous and 74 (60.7%) had multiple fibroids. The median interval between the initial and final examination was 21.5 (range, 8-90) months. The median fibroid volume gets higher by 35.2% per year. Small fibroids (< 20 mm mean diameter) grew significantly faster than larger fibroids (P = 0.007). The median grow bigger in size was significantly higher in cases of intramural fibroids (53.2 (interquartile range (IQR), 11.2-217)%) than in subserous fibroids (25.1 (IQR, 1.1-87.1)%) and submucous fibroids (22.8 (IQR, - 11.7 to 48.3)%) (P = 0.012). Multivariate analysis retained only fibroid size at presentation as an independent predictor of fibroid growth.

WHAT IS FIBROID?

Fibroids are non-cancerous growths that develop in or around the women womb (uterus). Their developments are made up of muscle and fibrous tissue, and diffrent in size. They're sometimes known as uterine myomas or leiomyomas. Most women do not know they
have fibroids because they don't have any symptoms.

Chapter Two

TYPES OF FIBROIDS

The medical term for fibroids is leiomyoma or myoma. The location, size and number of fibroids influence the severity of symptoms that a woman will experience. It is possible to have different type of fibroid at the same time if they grow in different parts of the reproductive system.

The main types of fibroids that can grow in a woman's body include*:*

Intramural fibroids — intramural fibroids are one the most common type of fibroid. They develop within the muscular uterine wall. If they're large enough, they can actually distort and stretch the uterus or womb. They can also affect in prolonged, heavy periods along with pressure and pain in the pelvic region.

Subserosal fibroids — Fibroids that develop outside the walls of the uterus sometimes press on the bladder, making urinary symptoms, i.e difficulty emptying your bladder. This type may also sometimes cause backaches. Backaches may happen when subserosal fibroids bulge from the back of your uterus and press on your spinal nerves, causing pressure in your back.

Penducluated fibroids — these fibroids develop on small stalks inside or outside of the uterus.

Submucosal fibroids — these developed just underneath the uterine lining. This type of fibroid is likely to cause heavy, prolonged menstrual bleeding. They can also sometimes gives problems to women trying to conceived. Submucosal tumors are not well known as other types.

Cervical fibroids — these develop in the cervical tissue, but they are rare compared to the other types of fibroids.

FAST FACT ON FIBROID

Here are some key points about fibroids.

- Fibroids are most common during the reproductive years.

- It is unclear exactly why they form, but they appear to grow when estrogen levels are higher.

- Most people experience no symptoms, but they can include lower backache, <u>constipation</u>, and excessive or painful uterine bleeding leading to anemia.

- Complications are rare, but they can be very serious.

- Fibroids are most often detected during a routine pelvic exam.

Chapter Three

WHAT ARE UTERINE FIBROIDS?

Fibroids are benign tumors comprises of smooth muscle cells and fibrous connective tissue. They grew in the uterus. According to research, It is estimated that 70-80% of women will develop fibroids in their lifetime—however, not every women will develop symptoms or require treatment. One of The most important features of fibroids is that they are not cancer, and they do not have the potential to become cancer. Due to that, it is reasonable for women that do not have symptoms to consider observation rather than cure. Research show us those fibroids grow at various rates, even in the same woman, and can be very close from the size of a pea to the size of a watermelon.

RISK FACTORS OF UTERINE FIBROIDS

- **Heredity**: A woman with a mother or sister who had/has fibroids is more likely to grow them herself.
- **Age**: Fibroids tend to show or occur when a woman is in her 30s and 40s.
- **Race**: African-American women are two to three times more likely to grow fibroids dthan women of other races or ethnicities. Black women have tendency to develop them at younger ages, and have more that are larger.
- **Diet**: Eating too much of poor quality beef and any type of pork is linked to higher fibroid risk.

- **Obesity**: Women who are overweight or obese are more likely to grow fibroids compared to women who maintain a healthy weight.
- **High Blood Pressure**: High blood pressure or hypertension tends to increase a woman's risk of fibroids.
- **Hypothyroidism**: Overt hypothyroidism has been identified with the presence of uterine leiomyomas (fibroids).
- **Early menstruation**: Women who start early menstruation prior to the age of 10 are at a higher risk for fibroids than women who started menstruating a little bit late after the age of 10.
- **Birth control**: Using birth control pills can make fibroids develop more quickly due to the high estrogen level in the body. Foods that are high in estrogen, and hormone-disrupting chemicals that mimic estrogen, may also play a major role in the growth of fibroids.

WHEN SURGERY IS NEEDED IN UTERINE FIBROID

Fibroid surgery might be recommended for women with strong symptoms, those women dealing with infertility, or those who are at high risk of dealing with complications during pregnancy or labor. Fibroid surgery is done BEFORE a woman is pregnant (not during pregnancy), since it can cause bleeding and other symptoms that would affect the pregnancy.

Uterine fibroid surgery can be done to inject fibroids only (this is called a myomectomy) or to inject a woman's entire uterus (called a hysterectomy). A hysterectomy is only suitable if a woman doesn't have an intension to become pregnant in the future, since her uterus is completely removed.

Before surgery is done a woman's medical personnel will likely try less invasive cure approaches, such as making use of birth control pills or hormone replacement drugs to reduced fibroid symptoms. Surgery is performed through either a small incision making use of laparoscopy, through the vagina, or through a larger incision into the abdominal region. The cure option called uterine fibroid embolization (UFE) is a reduced-invasive procedure that is making use of embolic agents to cover the arteries that provide blood to the fibroids, making them to shrink. UFE doesn't function for every type of fibroid and may also add to poor outcomes following the surgery.

SYMPTOMS OF FIBROIDS

Around 1- 3 women with fibroids will experience symptoms.

These may include:

- heavy, painful periods, also known as menorrhagia

- anemia from heavy periods

- lower backache or leg pain

- constipation

- discomfort in the lower abdomen, especially in the case of large fibroids

- frequent urination

- pain during intercourse, known as dyspareunia
  Other possible symptoms include:

- labor problems

- pregnancy problems

- fertility problems

- repeated miscarriages
  If fibroids are large, there may also be weight gain and
  swelling in the lower abdomen.

CAUSES OF FIBROIDS

It remains unknown exactly what causes fibroids. They
may be traced to estrogen levels.

During the reproductive years, estrogen
and progesterone levels increased.

When estrogen levels have increased, especially during
pregnancy, there is tendency for fibroid swell. They are
also more likely to grow when a woman is using a birth
control pills that contain estrogen.

Reduction in estrogen levels can cause fibroids may shrink, such during and after menopause.

Genetic factors are thought to affect the growth of fibroids. Having a close relative with fibroids increases the chance of developing them.

There is also a study that red meat, alcohol, and caffeine could high the risk of fibroids, and that a frequent intake of fruit and vegetables might reduce it.

NATURAL WAYS TO PREVENT FIBROIDS

Fibroids typically grow slowly or not at all. In many cases, they shrink on their own, especially after menopause. You may not need treatment unless you're bothered by symptoms. Your doctor will recommend the best treatment plan. You may need a combination of therapies.

In moderate to severe cases where symptoms are bothersome, worsening, or not improved with medication, fibroids may be treated with surgery or ultrasound therapy. Surgery may involve removing just the fibroids or your entire uterus.

At-home care, diet changes, and natural remedies may help treat fibroids and relieve symptoms. The lifestyle changes below are also important in the prevention of fibroids.

These natural treatments may or may not help your fibroid symptoms, since relief depends on how severe your symptoms are and how your fibroids have progressed. You should speak with your doctor before trying any of these options.

Weight loss

A clinical study in China showed that obesity and excess weight increased the risk for uterine fibroids. This happens because fat cells make high amounts of estrogen. Losing weight may help prevent or reduce the size of fibroids.

Nutrition

Your daily diet is a very important factor in treating fibroids. The right nutrition can help you maintain a healthy weight and reduce your risk. Certain foods can also help ease symptoms.

Foods to avoid

According to clinical studies, eating too much red meat increases your risk of uterine fibroids. Drinking alcohol also increases your risk.

Eating excess refined carbohydrates and sugary foods may trigger or worsen fibroids. These foods raise blood sugar levels. This causes your body to produce too much insulin hormone. Avoid or restrict simple refined carbohydrates like:

- white rice, pasta, and flour

- soda and other sugary drinks

- corn syrup

- boxed cereals

- baked goods (cakes, cookies, doughnuts)

- potato chips

- crackers

Foods to eat

Fiber-rich unprocessed foods help:

- curb your appetite

- balance hormones

- prevent excess weight gain

Brightly colored foods such as fruits and vegetables also help reduce inflammation and lower your risk for fibroids. Add these whole foods to your daily diet:

- raw and cooked vegetables and fruit

- dried fruit

- whole grains

- brown rice

- lentils and beans

- whole grain bread and pasta

- couscous

- quinoa

- fresh and dried herbs

Vitamins and supplements

Milk and dairy may help to reduce fibroids. Dairy products contain high amounts of calcium, magnesium, and phosphorus. These nutrients may help prevent growth of fibroids.

Some types of vitamins may also help reduce the growth and size of fibroids. Research confirms that your risk for fibroids may increase if you have low amounts of vitamin D and vitamin A from animal sources, such as dairy.

Uterine fibroids may worsen menstrual pain, bloating, and cramping. A number of vitamins may help ease these symptoms:

- vitamin B-1

- vitamin B-6

- vitamin E

- magnesium

- omega-3 fatty acids

You can find these vitamins in food as well as supplements. If you want to start incorporating supplements into your daily routine, talk with your doctor before you begin.

Blood pressure

A Dutch study found that there may be a link between high blood pressure and fibroids. Manage your blood pressure to help reduce your risk and improve your overall health:

- Limit foods with added salt or sodium.

- Check your blood pressure regularly and discuss readings with your doctor.

- Get regular exercise.

Herbal remedies

Herbal remedies may help to treat fibroids or reduce related symptoms. Further research is needed to find out if these remedies work and what the most effective dosage is.

Herbs are potent medicines and can interact with other drugs. They're also not regulated by the U.S. Food and Drug Administration. Talk with your doctor before taking herbal medicine.

Traditional Chinese Medicine

Herbal remedies are used in traditional Chinese Medicine to slow fibroid growth and treat symptoms. One herbal formula is called Guizhi fuling or Gui Zhi Fu Ling Tang. This formula contains several herbs that act to shrink uterine fibroids, balance hormone levels, and keep your uterus healthy:

- ramulus cinnamomi

- poria

- semen persicae

- radix paeoniae rubra

- radix paeoniae alba

- cortex moutan

Green tea

A bioflavonoid in green tea called EGCG may help reduce the size and number of fibroids. This may be due to its ability to reduce inflammation and remove toxins from your body.

Chasteberry

Chasteberry, or vitex, is taken for heavy menstrual bleeding, painful periods, and other symptoms. This herbal remedy helps to balance hormone levels.

Isphagula husk, senna, and castor oil

Fibrous herbs such as isphagula and senna are used as natural laxatives. Add these herbs to water or juice to help relieve constipation.

Castor oil is herbal oil that can be taken as a supplement to help occasional constipation.

Other remedies

At-home care may help to manage stress, which can worsen fibroids and your overall health. Try these treatment options that can help manage stress:

- warm compresses or applying local heat

- warm baths

- yoga and exercise

- massage therapy

Other treatment

In most cases, symptomatic fibroids are treated with hormonal medications, ultrasound therapy, surgery, and other treatment. Medications help to shrink fibroids or ease symptoms. Surgery may involve removing just the fibroids or your entire uterus.

Some treatments your doctor may recommend include:

- hormone balancing medications

- progestin-releasing intrauterine device (**IUD**)

- MRI-guided focused ultrasound surgery

- uterine artery embolization, which works by blocking blood supply to the fibroids and uterus

- myolysis, which is removal with radiofrequency waves

- cryomyolysis, which removes fibroids by freezing

- **myomectomy**, which is surgery to remove just fibroids

- hysterectomy, which surgically removes your uterus

Chapter Four

COMPLICATIONS

Fibroids do not normally result in complications, but if they happen, they can be very serious and even life-threatening.

Complications may include:

- **Menorrhagia**, also called heavy periods: This mostly prevent a woman from functioning normally during menstruation, causing depression, anemia, and fatigue.

- **Abdominal pain**: If fibroids are large, swelling and uncomfortable may happen in the lower abdomen. They may also bring about constipation with painful bowel movements.

- **Pregnancy problems**: Preterm birth, labor problems, and miscarriages may happen as estrogen levels rise significantly during pregnancy.

- **Infertility**: In most cases, fibroids can prevent the fertilized egg to attach itself to the lining of the womb. A submucosal fibroid developing on the inside of the uterine cavity may transform the shape of the womb, making conception more difficult.

- **Leiomyosarcoma**: This is a rare form of cancer that is thought by some to be able to grow inside of a fibroid in very critical cases.

Other serious complications include acute thromboembolism, deep vein thrombosis (DVT), acute renal failure, and internal bleeding.

A woman with fibroids who suddenly has a severe abdominal pain should contact her medical personnel immediately.

DIAGNOSIS

As fibroids often do not show symptoms, they are usually diagnosed during routine pelvic examinations.

The following diagnostic tests can detect fibroids and rule out other conditions:

- Medical personnel can create ultrasound images by scanning over the abdomen or by putting a small ultrasound probe into the vagina. Both approaches may be needed.

- An MRI can detect and determined the size and quantity of fibroids.

- A hysteroscopy uses a small device with a camera attached to the end to examine the inside of the womb. The device is inserted through the vagina and into the womb through the cervix. If necessary, the medical personnel can take a biopsy at the same time to identify potentially cancerous cells in the area.

A laparoscopy may also be done. In a laparoscopy, the medical personnel makes a small opening in the skin of the abdomen and puts a small tube with a lighted camera attached through the layers of abdominal wall. The camera reaches into the abdominopelvic cavity to examine the outside of the womb and its surrounding structures. If necessary, a biopsy can be taken from the outer layer of the womb.

FIBROID DURING PREGNANCY

When a woman has fibroids during pregnancy, what are some signs to look for or symptoms that might happen? Most times fibroids can cause complications during pregnancy and labor, and can cause a six-time greater risk of needing a cesarean section. They may also add to infertility if they are very serious. It may be difficult for an egg to become fertilized and then implant on the lining of the uterus when a large fibroid is present.

A woman's OB-GYN might recommend that she use medications prior to becoming pregnant in order to aid shrink fibroids. In serious cases surgery might also be performed before pregnancy, but it cannot be done once a woman is already pregnant because this can cause blood loss and pre-term labor. It's long been thought that fibroids high the risk of miscarriage during the first and second trimester. Morerover,, a new meta-analysis showed no sign of increase in spontaneous miscarriage risk among women with leiomyomas (fibroids) compared to those without.

It is possible that fibroids may high the risk for pre-term labor or complications during delivery including obstruction of the birth canal. However, not every woman with fibroids who becomes pregnant will experience any severe complications or symptoms.

Fibroids will increase in size during pregnancy because of high levels of estrogen. Bleeding and abdominal pain might also happen during pregnancy if the fibroid begins to lose its blood supply. A woman's medical personnel will likely recommend that she have more ultrasounds done during pregnancy than normal in order to monitor her fibroids.

Chapter Five

TREATMENT OF FIBROIDS

Treatment is only recommended for those women experiencing symptoms as a result of fibroids. If the fibroids are not affecting quality of life, cure may not be necessary.

Fibroids can cause heavy periods, but if these do not cause major problems, one may choose not to have treatment.

During menopause period, fibroids often shrink, and symptoms often become less apparent or even resolve completely.

When treatment is essential, it can take the form of medication or surgery. The location of the fibroids, the seriousness of the symptoms, and any future childbearing plans can all affect the decision.

Medication

The first line of treatment for fibroids is medication.

A drug known as a gonadotropin-releasing hormone agonist (GnRHa) affect the body to produce less estrogen and progesterone. This shrinks fibroids. GnRHa ends the

menstrual cycle without affecting fertility after the end of
treatment.

GnRH agonists can cause menopause-like symptoms,
including hot flashes, a tendency to sweat more, vaginal
dryness, and, in most cases, increased the risk
of osteoporosis.

They may be given before surgery to shrink the fibroids.
The drug is for short-term use only.

Other drugs may be used, but they may be less effective
when treating larger fibroids.

These include:

- **Non-steroidal anti-inflammatory drugs (NSAIDs)**:
  These comprises of mefenamic and ibuprofen, which is
  available to buy in the drug store. Anti-inflammatory
  medications lower the production of hormone-like lipid
  compounds called prostaglandins. Prostaglandins are
  known with crampy periods, and they are thought to be
  associated with heavy menstrual periods. For those with
  fibroids, an NSAID may be effective at reducing fibroid
  pain, does not reduce bleeding from fibroids, and does
  not affect fertility.

- **Birth control pills**: Oral contraceptives help to normalize the ovulation cycle, and they may aid in reducing the amount of pain or bleeding during periods.

- **Levonorgestrel intrauterine system (LNG-IUS)**: This is a plastic device which is placed inside the womb. It then allowed a hormone called levonorgestrel over an extended timeframe. The hormone stops the inside lining of the womb from developing too fast, which lower menstrual bleeding. Serious effects include irregular bleeding for up to 6 months or longer, headaches, breast tenderness, and acne. In some cases, it can stop periods.

Surgery

Serious fibroids may not respond to more conservative curing options, and surgery may be necessary.

The treating medical personnel may consider the following procedures:

- **Hysterectomy**: A hysterectomy is the partial or total removal of the womb. This action is required for treating extremely large fibroids or too much of bleeding. A total hysterectomy can stop the return of fibroids. If a surgeon also takes off the ovaries and fallopian tubes, this can lead to reduction of libido and early menopause.

- **Myomectomy**: This is the take- off of fibroids from the muscular wall of the womb. It can assist women who still want to bear children. Women with large fibroids, or fibroids located in particular parts of their womb, may not be favour by this surgery.

- **Endometrial ablation**: Eliminating the lining inside of the womb may assist if fibroids are near the inner surface of the womb. Endometrial ablation may be an effective alternative to a hysterectomy for most women with fibroids.

- **Uterine artery embolization (UAE), more specifically uterine fibroid embolization (UFE)**: Taking off the blood supply to the area shrinks the fibroid. Guided by fluoroscopic X-ray imaging, a chemical is injected through a catheter into the arteries supplying blood to any fibroids. This process lowers or removes symptoms in up to 90% of people living with fibroids but is not good for women who are pregnant and typically not for those who still wish to bear children.

- **MRI-guided percutaneous laser ablation**: An MRI scan is used to detect the fibroids. Fine needles are then put through the skin and body tissues of the patient and pushed until they reach the targeted fibroids. A laser fiber device is put through the needles. A laser light is sent through the device to shrink the fibroids.

- **MRI-guided focused ultrasound surgery**: An MRI scan detects the fibroids, and high energy ultrasound waves are delivered to shrink them.

EFFECTS OF FIBROID

Fibroids usually don't have any other negative effects aside from the symptoms already described and the associated problems. But most women worry that fibroids may impact in their fertility. This is only true of certain types of fibroids. Professional estimates that only 1 to 2% of infertility cases are caused by fibroids. Most women diagonised with fibroids can still become pregnant.

Fibroids that develop just under the lining of the womb are particularly likely to disrupt the function of the womb – for example by stopping fertilized egg cells from attaching. Fibroids that develop on the outside of the womb probably don't affect fertility. It is not well known whether fibroids in the wall of the womb can cause fertility.

Fibroids also don't usually high the risk of complications during pregnancy. It is generally believed that only fibroids in the wall of the womb and under the lining of the womb may increase the risk of miscarriage. Fibroids in general probably hardly affect the risk of a baby being born too soon. A fibroid that is reduced in the womb may prevent the baby's head from entering the lower pelvis during birth, making a Cesarean section necessary.

Most women worry that fibroids might turn cancerous, but this fear is not justified. Fibroids are not cancerous.

People used to think that fibroids could grow into cancerous tumors in connective tissue (sarcoma) in extremely serious cases, but there is no scientific proof to support this.

FREQUENTLY ASKED QUESTION ON FIBROID

What is a uterine fibroid?
Uterine fibroids are growths that form inside the lining of the uterus, on its outer surface, within its wall, or attached by a stem-like structure. They are typically benign.

Do all women develop uterine fibroids?
Out of the entire population of women, approximately 60-80% of women will have fibroids by the time menopause is reached.

What causes uterine fibroids?
The cause of fibroids is not well known but the hormone estrogen seems to make them develop. Due to the highest levels of estrogen are produced during a women's childbearing years, most women are affected in their 30's and 40's. Fibroids are rare in women under 20, and they typically stabilize in size or shrink after menopause.

Are there risk factors for uterine fibroids?
A family history of fibroids, obesity, or early onset of
puberty cans high the risk of women developing uterine
fibroids.

Do all uterine fibroids need treatment?
Most fibroids do not cause any symptoms and you may
choose to do nothing. Surgical intervention is required in
~20% of women with fibroids. Cure for fibroids might be
necessary when they cause:

- Long, gushing periods and cramping
- Spotting or bleeding between periods
- Painful periods
- An urge to urinate often
- Pain during sex
- Lower back pain
- Pelvic pain
- Difficulty getting pregnant
- Problems during pregnancy, such as miscarriage or
  preterm labor
- Constipation and backache
- Fullness or pressure in your belly

How are uterine fibroids diagnosed?
The diagnosis of uterine fibroids can often be done
through a pelvic exam. Your medical personnel may send
you to have an ultrasound or another type of test that
shows pictures of your uterus. These assist your medical
personnel see how large your fibroids are and where they
are developing.

Will I have to have surgery for a uterine fibroid?
Not all fibroids need intervention. In most cases, such as
large fibroids, or when a woman is experiencing
infertility, it may be necessary to surgically take off the
uterine fibroid(s). Your medical personnel will discuss all
options with you.

About the **Author**

Dr. Bayo is a pastor and a medical practioner who studied pharmacy in SefakoMakgatho Health Sciences University (SMU) in South Africa and receive his Phd in Lipscomb University in Missouri-columbia.
He has involved himself into prescriptions and cure of diseases and sickness. He is a solution to many problems amidst its environment such has cancer, stroke infection, erectile dysfuntion, anti-biotic infection, how to reduce your blood pressure and lots more to mention but a little. He has been eagerly and greatly having impact in the life of msny others in the area of pharmaceutical trainings and has been building people to be pharmaceutically awake in order not to be deceived by fake drug sellers out there.
Other books by Dr. Bayo are: 100% ways to stay healthy with Moringa, 100% natural ways to treat leukemia , Natural ways to treat erectile dysfunction in men and Basic facts about coronavirus and it,s prevention.

Acknowledgments

My appreciation goes to God, Almighty for the opportunity to collate this manuscript, and for wisdom he gave me to spread the knowledge around. Also I appreciate everyone that supported me during the compilation, proof reading and publishing of the book

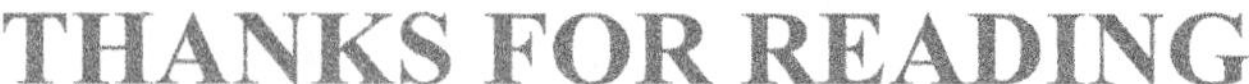

THANKS FOR READING

www.ingramcontent.com/pod-product-compliance
Lightning Source LLC
Chambersburg PA
CBHW071500150726
48000CB00006B/2643